HEMATOLOGY SELF-ASSESSMENT SERIES: WHITE BLOOD CELL DISORDERS

Dr. Bhratri Bhushan
MBBS, MD (internal medicine), DM (medical oncology)
Consultant medical oncologist and hematologist

This work is provided "as is," and the author and the publisher disclaim any and all warranties, express or implied, including any warranties as to accuracy, comprehensiveness, or currency of the content of this work. This work is no substitute for individual patient assessment based on healthcare professionals' examination of each patient and consideration of, among other things, age, weight, gender, current or prior medical conditions, medication history, labora-tory data, and other factors unique to the patient. The publisher does not provide medical advice or guidance, and this work is merely a reference tool. Healthcare professionals, and not the publisher, are solely responsible for the use of this work including all medical judgments and for any resulting diagno-sis and treatments. Given continuous, rapid advances in medical science and health information, independent professional verification of medical diagnoses, indications, appropriate pharmaceutical selections and dosages, and treatment options should be made and healthcare professionals should consult a variety of sources. When prescribing medication, healthcare professionals are advised to consult the product information sheet (the manufacturer's package insert) accompanying each drug to verify, among other things, conditions of use, warn-ings, and side effects and identify any changes in dosage schedule or contraindi-cations, particularly if the medication to be administered is new, infrequently used, or has a narrow therapeutic range. To the maximum extent permitted under applicable law, no responsibility is assumed by the publisher for any injury and/or damage to persons or property as a matter of products liability, negligence law or otherwise, or from any reference to or use by any person of this work.

CONTENTS

PROPHYLAXIS AND MANAGEMENT OF 83
NEUTROPENIA

Dedicated to my father Dr. Bharat Bhushan

PREFACE

This book covers the topics of nonmalignant white blood cell disorders in an interactive, self-assessment format. Topics like white blood cell biology, lab hematology pertinent to white blood cells, Langerhans cell histiocytosis, hemophagocytic lymphohistiocytosis, congenital disorders, iatrogenic neutropenia and leukopenia, CHIP, ICUS, CCUS, neutropenia and its management et cetera are covered in depth.

Malignant white blood cell disorders are not covered in this book and the review of malignant hematology conditions can be found in the book, Oncology MCQs for NEET-SS, vol. 2 by the author (available at https://www.amazon.in/dp/B083VXXZY8)

ABOUT THE AUTHOR

Dr. Bhratri Bhushan MBBS, MD (Internal medicine), DM (Medical oncology) is a consultant medical oncologist and hematologist. He has published over twenty books on the subject of oncology and his papers have been published in renowned journals of medical literature. Many of his books have been bestsellers. His works can be found at his authorcental page: https://www.amazon.com/-/e/B07RC35JKX

BIOLOGY

Q. All of the following are true except:
1. Stem cell factor is also known as Steel factor
2. G-CSF is essential for the amplification and terminal differentiation of neutrophil progenitors and precursors
3. M-CSF/CSF1 is a monocyte lineage specific factor
4. IL-12 is an eosinophil lineage specific factor

Answer: IL-12 is an eosinophil lineage specific factor
In fact, **IL-5** is an eosinophil lineage specific factor.

Q. Which of the following points is wrong regarding development of myeloid lineage cells:
1. Myeloblasts are the earliest myeloid precursors recognizable by light microscopy
2. Promyelocytes are larger than myeloblasts with their size being > 20 microns

3. Myelocytes are the last precursor capable of undergoing cell division
4. Promyelocytes are characterized by secondary or azurophilic granules

Answer: Promyelocytes are characterized by secondary or azurophilic granules

In fact, promyelocytes are characterized by primary or azurophilic granules.

Q. Which of the following is not a feature of bands:
1. They have elongated, horseshoe-shaped nuclei
2. The ratio of azurophilic primary granules to specific secondary granules is approximately 1:2 in these cells
3. Tertiary (gelatinase) granules are not present
4. These are fully functional phagocytes

Answer: Tertiary (gelatinase) granules are not present

In fact, tertiary granules are present.

To clarify the fourth option, the bands are fully functional and they are included in the absolute neutrophil count (ANC).

Q. Which of the following is not a feature of PMNs:
1. They are of variable size with average diameter being 20 microns
2. Their nucleus has three lobes on average
3. Approximately 3 percent of PMNs from females have a visible Barr body which is an inactivated X chromosome
4. They show peroxidase-positive primary granules and peroxidase-negative secondary granules

Answer: They are of variable size with average diameter being 20 microns

The fact is that PMNs are of consistently similar size and the average diameter is 13 microns.

Q. The maturation time for neutrophils from the myeloblast stage is:
1. 1 day
2. 8 days
3. 14 days
4. 28 days

Answer: 8 days

Q. What is the mean lifespan of neutrophils:
1. 5-8 days

2. 1-2 days
3. 10-14 days
4. More than a month

Answer: 5-8 days

Notes on fate of monocytes:
Monocytes differentiate further into fixed-tissue macrophages, including:

1. Alveolar macrophages
2. Hepatic Kupffer cells
3. Dermal Langerhans' cells
4. Osteoclasts
5. Peritoneal and pleural macrophages
6. Brain microglial cells (controversial)

Q. Human pulmonary alveolar proteinosis (PAP) is caused by:

1. Autoantibodies to GM-CSF
2. Autoantibodies to G-CSF
3. Autoantibodies to erythropoietin
4. Autoantibodies to stem cell factor

Answer: Autoantibodies to GM-CSF

LAB HEMATOLOGY

Notes on some formulas:
1. Mean corpuscular volume (MCV; in femto-liters [fL]) = 10 x HCT (percent) ÷ RBC (millions/microL)
2. Mean corpuscular hemoglobin (MCH; in picograms [pg]/red cell) = HGB (g/dL) x 10 ÷ RBC (millions/microL)
3. Mean corpuscular hemoglobin concentration (MCHC), in grams per deciliter (g/dL) = HGB (g/dL) X 100 ÷ HCT (percent)
4. Hematocrit = (RBC x MCV)/10

Q. In which of the following conditions RDW is only slightly elevated:
1. Iron deficiency
2. Transfused anemia
3. Myelodysplastic syndrome
4. Thalassemia trait

Answer: thalassemia trait

In the other three conditions, RDW is **very** elevated. In anemia of chronic disease, RDW is slightly elevated.

Q. Use of which of the following agents during collection of peripheral blood is most commonly associated with pseudothrombocytopenia:

1. EDTA
2. Heparin
3. Sodium citrate
4. Dimethyl sulfoxide

Answer: EDTA

Q. Which of the following statements is correct:

1. Blood samples be kept at room temperature if analysis is to occur within eight hours of collection
2. Blood samples should be refrigerated if the analysis is to occur up to 24 hours after collection
3. Samples more than 36 hours old should not be used for CBC testing
4. All of the above

Answer: all of the above

Q. In Coulter instruments, when taking readings about RBCs, a left "shoulder" extension to the curve indicates presence of what:

1. Schistocytes
2. Sideroblasts
3. Reticulocytes
4. RBC agglutinins

Answer: schistocytes

Notes on abnormalities of RBC distribution on Coulter instruments:

1. A left "shoulder" extension to the curve, or failure of the curve to reach baseline on the left side is due to RBCs with smaller volumes. It can be seen when microspherocytes or schistocytes are present. It may also be seen when platelet clumps or macrothrombocytes.
2. A separate RBC population to the left can indicate the presence of two populations of red cells, as seen in X-linked sideroblastic anemia.
3. A right-sided shoulder usually corresponds to a population of extremely large RBCs (macrocytes) or reticulocytes.
4. A trailing erythrocyte population to the extreme right can indicate the presence of RBC agglutinins.

Q. Platelets with a higher MPV are expected to be seen in:

1. Destructive thrombocytopenia

2. Marrow hypoplasia
3. Marrow aplasia
4. All of the above

Answer: Destructive thrombocytopenia

Higher MPV is seen when destruction of platelets is there but marrow is active as in immune thrombocytopenia [ITP]. It is also seen in some congenital thrombocytopenias like gray platelet syndrome, May-Hegglin anomaly, and Bernard-Soulier syndrome.

Low MPV is seen when marrow is not active enough, like in aplastic anemia. It is also seen in Wiskott-Aldrich syndrome.
In hypersplenism platelets with low MPV are seen whereas in hyposplenic states platelets with higher MPV are seen.

Q. In instruments of hematology using scattered light for cell counting, the light is measured at low and high forward angles. How much is the low forward angle in these machines:
1. 0 to 3 degrees
2. 5 to 15 degrees
3. 15 to 30 degrees
4. 30 to 45 degrees

Answer: 0 to 3 degrees

Q. Which is the proposed international reference method for enumeration of platelets:

1. Immunologic method
2. Coulter method
3. Light scattering method
4. There is no consensus in this regard

Answer: immunologic method

CD61 monoclonal antibody is used for this. Another antibody is CD41a.

Q. While performing the differential leukocyte count by suspension method, the smallest size group of cells is:

1. Lymphocytes
2. Eosinophils
3. Band neutrophils
4. Monocytes

Answer: lymphocytes

These values are slightly different than the ones we usually memorize. In the "three-part differential" there are three groups of cells:

1. Lymphocytes and basophils are the smallest size group (35 to 90 fL)
2. Segmented and band neutrophils and eo-

sinophils ("granulocytes") in the largest size group (>160 fL)

3. Monocytes and other mononuclear cells, including immature granulocytes and a portion of the eosinophils, are found in a smaller intermediate size peak between 90 and 160 fL

There are also five-part differential machines that report the basic five leukocyte subsets (neutrophils, eosinophils, basophils, lymphocytes, and monocytes) and also, seven part differential machines that add quantification of immature granulocytes and nucleated red blood cells to the five-part differential.

The current generation of instruments use the following techniques to produce a final DLC report:

1. Impedance volume with direct current (DC)
2. Radiofrequency (RF) conductivity (with impedance aperture)
3. Laser light scattering
4. Peroxidase staining
5. Propidium iodide fluorescence (for nucleated RBC and non-viable cells)
6. Cell-specific lysing reagents
7. Polymethine RNA/DNA histone dye
8. Digital imaging

Q. Which of the following is not a cause of spurious increase in MCHC:
1. A spuriously elevated HGB
2. A spuriously high RBC count
3. Lipemia
4. A very high WBC count

Answer: A spuriously high RBC count

In fact, it is the spuriously low RBC count that leads to spurious increases in MCHC. Apart from the three situations listed above, other causes of a spuriously high MCHC are presence of a precipitating monoclonal protein and presence of a cold agglutinin.

On the other hand, causes of spuriously decreased MCHC are:
1. Iron deficiency anemia
2. Hyperglycemia (it leads to temporary changes in readings)

Q. Peripheral smear examination offers many insights and is a cheap method. Which of the following is not true about a peripheral smear examination:
1. The thick of the slide may be useful in searching for the presence of malarial parasites
2. The thin end of the slide may be useful for identifying Auer rods

3. The thick end of the slide is more useful in identification of circulating tumor cells
4. None of the above

Answer: The thick end of the slide is more useful in identification of circulating tumor cells

In fact, CTCs are better visualized in the thick end.

Q. RBC rouleaux formation is seen in all except:
1. Multiple myeloma
2. Decreased levels of fibrinogen
3. Polyclonal gammopathy
4. Monoclonal gammopathy

Answer: decreased level of fibrinogen

In fact, increased levels of fibrinogen are associated with rouleaux formation.

Q. Which of the following is not true about the normal red cells:
1. They are the second most abundant cells in the peripheral smear
2. They are approximate the size of the lymphocyte nucleus
3. Their diameter is 7 to 8 microns
4. Their mean corpuscular volume (MCV) of approximately 90 femtoliters

Answer: They are the second most abundant cells in the peripheral smear

In fact, they are **the most** abundant cells in the peripheral smear.

Q. RBCs are generally round and have a smooth surface. Changes in their shape are known as poikilocytosis. Which of the following is not a correct statement in this regard:
1. Macroovalocytes suggest deficiency of vitamin B12 or folic acid
2. Schistocytes or helmet shaped cells are seen in idiopathic thrombocytopenic purpura
3. Teardrop-shaped red cells are seen in primary myelofibrosis
4. Teardrop shaped cells may be seen in thalassemia

Answer: Schistocytes or helmet shaped cells are seen in idiopathic thrombocytopenic purpura
In fact, schistocytes are seen in thrombotic thrombocytopenic purpura

Q. Approximately what fraction of area of red cell should appear clear on light microscopy:
1. 0%

2. 33%
3. 50%
4. 66%

Answer: 33%

This clear area is in the form of central pallor and occupies one-third of the red cell.

When hemoglobin concentration is low, this area is increased in size and in conditions like hereditary spherocytosis and autoimmune hemolytic anemia, this area is lost.

Q. Metamyelocytes and myelocytes may be seen in peripheral circulation during:
1. Infections
2. Pregnancy
3. Leukemoid reactions
4. They are never seen in nonmalignant conditions

Answer: first three options are correct

That being said, it's not usual for them to appear in the peripheral circulation in the above mentioned conditions but they may be seen. On the other hand cells like promyelocytes and myeloblasts are almost exclusively seen in hematologic malignancies.

Q. Leuko-erythroblastic blood picture is defined as the combined presence of all of the following except:
1. Early neutrophil forms
2. Nucleated red blood cells
3. Megakaryocytes
4. Teardrop-shaped red blood cells

Answer: megakaryocytes

This picture is suggestive of bone marrow invasion and/or fibrosis.

Q. A leukemic hiatus is frequently seen in CML patients, which means:
1. There is a greater percent of myelocytes than metamyelocytes in the peripheral blood
2. There is a lesser percent of myelocytes than metamyelocytes in the peripheral blood
3. There is a greater percent of meta-myelocytes than myelocytes in the bone marrow
4. There is a lesser percent of meta-myelocytes than myelocytes in the bone marrow

Answer: There is a greater percent of myelocytes than metamyelocytes in the peripheral blood

Q. Increased lobulation of neutrophils, known as hyperlobulation, is seen in all except:
1. Vitamin B12 deficiency
2. Iron deficiency anemia
3. Heat stroke
4. Myelodysplastic syndrome

Answer: myelodysplastic syndrome

In MDS, there is reduced lobulation of matured neutrophils known as the pseudo-Pelger-Huet anomaly. In the Pelger-Huet anomaly too, hypolobulation is seen. The abnormal cells in these two disorders have bilobed nucleus connected by a thin strand, giving a "pince-nez" appearance.

Q. In Chediak-Higashi syndrome, which abnormality of neutrophils is seen:
1. Increased lobulation
2. Giant cytoplasmic granules
3. Reduced or absent toxic granules in cases of infection
4. Recurrent pyogenic infection with neutrophil abnormalities

Answer: Reduced or absent toxic granules in cases of

infection

This syndrome is characterized by giant cytoplasmic granules within neutrophils.

Dohle bodies are light blue colored, situated near the periphery and seen in neutrophils of patients with infection.

Q. Which of the following is the least common circulating white blood cell:

1. Eosinophil
2. Basophil
3. Monocyte
4. Neutrophil

Answer: basophils.

They constitute less than 1% of total circulating white cell population.

Basophilia is seen in myeloproliferative disorders, hypersensitivity or inflammatory reactions, hypothyroidism (myxedema), and certain infections.

Q. Which are the largest normal cells seen on a peripheral blood smear;

1. Monocytes
2. Basophils

3. Reticulocytes
4. Lymphocytes

Answer: monocytes

Q. Large platelets may be seen in:
1. Disseminated intravascular coagulation
2. Thrombotic thrombocytopenic purpura
3. Hemolytic uremic syndrome (HUS)
4. All of the above

Answer: all of the above

Drug-induced thrombotic microangiopathy (DITMA) is also a cause.

Q. Microcytosis (of RBCs) in an adult may be seen in:
1. Iron deficiency
2. Thalassemia
3. Sideroblastic anemias
4. Chronic copper toxicity

Answer: chronic copper toxicity

The first three are recognized causes of microcytosis.

Chronic lead poisoning is another known cause of microcytosis.

Q. Polychromatophilia is typical of:
1. Basophils
2. Eosinophils
3. Reticulocytes
4. Band forms

Answer: reticulocytes

Notes on shapes of RBCs:
1. Bite cells are seen in hemolytic anemia, especially G6PD. The rigid precipitates of denatured hemoglobin are known as Heinz bodies
2. In sickle cell anemia, the RBCs (obviously) look like sickles; other words are "canoe-like" or "pita bread-like".
3. Target cells have a "bull's eye" extra drop of hemoglobin in their center. They are seen in obstructive liver disease, postsplenec-tomy states, and hemoglobinopathies such as thalassemia and Hb C.
4. Echinocytes/burr cells/crenated cells are seen most commonly in uremia.
5. Acanthocytes or spur cells are seen in liver disease.
6. Teardrop-shaped red cells are are seen in primary myelofibrosis and thalassemic disorders.

Q. Nucleated red blood cells are seen in the peripheral blood in all of the following conditions except:

1. Severe hemolysis
2. Myelofibrosis
3. Profound stress
4. Severe iron deficiency anemia

Answer: Severe iron deficiency anemia

Q. Which of the following is not true:

1. Howell-Jolly bodies are nuclear remnants within red cells seen in hypersplenism
2. Heinz bodies are aggregates of denatured hemoglobin, found in G6PD deficient subjects
3. Basophilic stippling occurs due to ribosome precipitates and seen in thalassemias and lead poisoning
4. Pappenheimer bodies are iron-containing dark blue granules found in red cells in patients with sideroblastic anemia

Answer: Howell-Jolly bodies are nuclear remnants within red cells seen in hypersplenism

Howell-Jolly bodies are seen in patients with either absence of spleen or reduced function of spleen (like in cases of surgical removal of the spleen and in sickle cell anemia, when the crisis lead to infarction of spleen.

Q. The infectious agent most commonly leading to "red cell ghosts" is:
1. Clostridium perfringens
2. Staphylococcus aureus
3. Haemophilus influenzae
4. Neisseria meningitidis

Answer: Clostridium perfringens

Q. The formula for calculation of absolute neutrophil count is:
1. ANC = WBC (cells/microL) x percent (PMNs + bands) ÷ 100
2. ANC = WBC (cells/microL) x percent (PMNs + multinucleated cells) ÷ 100
3. ANC = WBC (cells/microL) x percent (PMNs + bands)
4. ANC = WBC (cells/microL) x percent (PMNs) ÷ 100

Answer: ANC = WBC (cells/microL) x percent (PMNs + bands) ÷ 100

The point to remember here is that bands are considered functional neutrophils.

Q. In which of the following condition will the production of neutrophils will not be decreased:
1. Severe congenital neutropenia
2. Shwachman-Diamond syndrome
3. Chediak Higashi syndrome
4. None of the above

Answer: none of the above

In all of the above mentioned conditions the production of neutrophils will be decreased.

Other causes of decreased neutrophil production are aplastic anemia, paroxysmal nocturnal hemoglobinuria (PNH) etc.

Q. Chronic granulomatous disease is due to defects in:
1. NADPH oxidase
2. NADPH reductase
3. NADPH transcriptase
4. NADPH reuptake

Answer: NADPH oxidase

Defects in NADPH oxidase result in an inability of neutrophils to make superoxide.

This disease is most of the times X-linked and affects only males. In rare cases females may suffer from a mild form of CGD.

The diagnosis of CGD is established by showing absence of the ability to make superoxide in response to stimulation with phorbol myristate acetate (PMA). Superoxide production is indirectly assayed as an inability to reduce dihydrorhodamine (DHR) to its fluorescent form (which can be assayed using flow cytometry) or to reduce nitroblue tetrazolium (NBT), which is assayed using the NBT slide test.

Q. Leukocyte adhesion deficiency I is caused by:
1. Absence of the transmembrane protein CD18
2. Absence of the transmembrane protein CD28
3. Increased levels of the transmembrane protein CD18
4. Increased levels of the transmembrane protein CD18

Answer: Absence of the transmembrane protein CD18

On the other hand LAD-II is caused by decreased sialyl-Lewis-X on the neutrophil surface.

Q. Which of the following is not a feature of Chediak-Higashi syndrome:

1. Partial albinism
2. Nystagmus
3. Defects in chemotaxis
4. Absence of granules visible in the peripheral blood smear

Answer: Absence of granules visible in the peripheral blood smear

In fact, a feature of this syndrome is the presence of huge granules in the peripheral blood smear.

Q. Hyperimmunoglobulin E syndrome results i defects in neutrophil function due to mutations in:
1. STAT 3
2. JAK 1
3. BRAF
4. NADPH oxidase

Answer: STAT 3

This syndrome is also known as Job syndrome.

Q. The definition of lymphocytosis in an adult is:
1. >4000 lymphocytes/microL in the peripheral blood
2. >8000 lymphocytes/microL in the peripheral blood
3. >2000 lymphocytes/microL in the periph-

eral blood
4. >1000 lymphocytes/microL in the peripheral blood

Answer: >4000 lymphocytes/microL in the peripheral blood

Q. The definition of lymphocytopenia in an adult is:
1. <4000 lymphocytes/microL in the peripheral blood
2. <8000 lymphocytes/microL in the peripheral blood
3. <1500 lymphocytes/microL in the peripheral blood
4. <1000 lymphocytes/microL in the peripheral blood

Answer: <1000 lymphocytes/microL in the peripheral blood

It should be noted that these values are not absolute and some flexibility is allowed in interpretation.

Formula for calculation of absolute lymphocyte count (ALC) (cells/microL) = WBC (cells/microL) x percent lymphocytes ÷ 100

Q. In the peripheral blood, the most abundant

lymphocyte population is of:
1. T cells
2. B cells
3. NK cells
4. All of the above are found in almost equal numbers

Answer: T cells

T cells are 60 to 80 percent, B cells are 10 to 20 percent and NK cells are 5 to 10 percent of total peripheral blood lymphocytes.

Around 66% of T cells are CD4+ cells and 33% are CD8+ cells.

Q. Lymphocytosis is associated with:
1. *B. pertussis* infection
2. *B. parapertussis* infection
3. Both of the above
4. None of the above

Answer: *B. pertussis* infection

Q. All of the following are associated with lymphocytopenia except:
1. Wiskott-Aldrich syndrome
2. HIV infection
3. Protein energy malnutrition

    4. EBV infection

Answer: EBV infection

In fact, EBV infection is **characterized** by lymphocytosis.

Drugs frequently associated with drug reaction with eosinophilia and systemic symptoms (DRESS):
1. Allopurinol
2. Carbamazepine, lamotrigine, phenytoin
3. Vancomycin, minocycline, dapsone, sulfamethoxazole

Notes on congenital causes of pancytopenia:
1. Wiskott Aldrich syndrome
2. Fanconi anemia
3. Dyskeratosis congenita/telomere biology disorders
4. Shwachman-Diamond syndrome
5. GATA2 deficiency
6. Hemophagocytic lymphohistiocytosis (HLH)

Q. The most accepted definition of neutropenia in adults in a neutrophil count in the peripheral blood of:
1. <1500 cells/microL
2. <2000 cells/microL

     3. <1000 cells/microL
     4. <500 cells/microL

Answer: <1500 cells/microL

It should be remembered that this value, and other such values, are not absolute and different institutes and organizations have different definitions; like the World Health Organization uses ANC of ≤1800 cells/microL to define neutropenia.

Notes on categories of neutropenia:
     1. Mild: ANC ≥1000 and <1500 cells/microL
     2. Moderate: ANC ≥500 and <1000 cells/microL
     3. Severe: ANC <500 cells/microL
     4. Agranulocytosis: ANC <200 cells/microL

Q. The most common cause of neutropenia is:
     1. Infections
     2. Medications
     3. Nutritional
     4. Familial

Answer: medications

Rheumatologic disorders are also a common and important cause of neutropenia.

Q. In immunocompromised patients, the chest radiograph appearance of Pneumocystis jirovecii infection is:
1. Nodular infiltrates
2. Diffuse interstitial infiltrates
3. Basal infiltrates
4. Pleural effusion with patchy consolidation

Answer: Diffuse interstitial infiltrates

In viral infections, ARDS etc. too, there are diffuse interstitial infiltrates.

Q. Which of the following is not true about benign ethnic neutropenia:
1. It is an inherited cause of mild/moderate neutropenia
2. It is associated with increased risk for infections
3. It is more prevalent in people of African descent
4. It has been described in up to 25 to 40 percent of individuals of African origin

Answer: It is associated with increased risk for infections

Note the word "benign" in it. The risk of infections is not increased.

It is associated with a single nucleotide polymorphism (SNP) of the *ACKR1* gene.

Q. Patients with benign ethnic neutropenia are usually:
1. Duffy null
2. O negative and Rh negative
3. Of Bombay blood group
4. Of unclassifiable blood group type

Answer: Duffy null

HEMOPHAGOCYTIC LYMPHOHISTIOCYTOSIS

Q. Hemophagocytic lymphohistiocytosis most frequently affects which population:
1. Infants
2. Early adolescence
3. Late adulthood
4. Elderly

Answer: infants

HLH is a life-threatening syndrome of excessive immune activation. It most frequently affects infants from birth to 18 months of age.

The highest incidence in those <3 months.

HLH is broadly of two types: primary and secondary. Primary HLH is caused by a gene mutation, either at one of the FHL loci or in a gene responsible for one of several immunodeficiency syndromes. Secondary HLH cases have **no** known familial mutation.

Macrophage activation syndrome is a form of HLH, which is often associated with juvenile rheumatologic diseases.

Q. Which of the following is true about pathogenesis and prognostic factors in HLH:
1. In HLH, macrophages become activated and secrete excessive amounts of cytokines
2. In HLH, NK cells fail to eliminate activated macrophages
3. In HLH, increased CD8 numbers and decreased CD4/CD8 ratios is associated with worse survival
4. Decreased total CD3 numbers is associated with a bad outcome

Answer: In HLH, increased CD8 numbers and decreased CD4/CD8 ratios is associated with worse survival

In fact, in HLH, increased CD8 numbers and decreased CD4/CD8 ratios is associated with **better** survival outcomes.

Q. Hemophagocytosis is frequently observed in HLH. Macrophage cytoplasm should show which kinds of cells or their fragments, to be categorized as hemophagocytosis:
1. Red blood cells
2. Platelets

3. White blood cells
4. Any of the above

Answer: any of the above

Q. Unbound (free) IL-18 levels are higher in:
1. Macrophage activation syndrome
2. Familial HLH
3. The levels are not elevated in either MAS or HLH
4. The levels are elevated to the same degree in both MAS and HLH

Answer: MAS

Unbound IL-18 level >24,000 pg/mL could distinguish MAS from familial HLH.

Q. Which is the most common infectious trigger for development of HLH:
1. EBV
2. HSV
3. HIV
4. CMV

Answer: EBV

Patients with X-linked lymphoproliferative disease (XLP) are at particularly high risk.

Interestingly, immune checkpoint inhibitors **may be** linked to the development of HLH.

Q. The genes for which cellular mechanisms are most commonly affected in HLH:
    1. Perforin-dependent cytotoxicity
    2. Antibody dependent cytotoxicity
    3. Complement cascade
    4. Cell energetics and anaerobic metabolism

Answer: Perforin-dependent cytotoxicity

Many HLH gene mutations map to loci that code for elements of the cytotoxic granule formation and release pathway, and have been labeled familial hemophagocytic lymphohistiocytosis (FHL) loci. The most important of these are:
    1. PRF1/Perforin (FHL2)
    2. UNC13D/Munc13-4 (FHL3)
    3. STX11/Syntaxin 11 (FHL4)
    4. STXBP2/Munc18-2 (FHL5)

Q. Which of the following immunodeficiency syndromes is least likely to be associated with increased incidence of HLH:
    1. Griscelli syndrome
    2. Chediak-Higashi syndrome
    3. Severe combined immunodeficiency

4. X-linked immunoproliferative disease

Answer: severe combined immunodeficiency

Notes on immunodeficiency syndromes associated with HLH:

1. Griscelli syndrome is caused by mutations of *RAB27A*

2. Chediak-Higashi syndrome is caused by mutations of *CHS1/LYST*. It is characterized by partial oculocutaneous albinism, neutrophil defects, neutropenia, and neurologic abnormalities.

3. X-linked lymphoproliferative disease is caused by mutations in SH2 domain protein 1A (*SH2D1A*).

4. XMEN disease: **X**-linked immunodeficiency with **m**agnesium defect, **E**BV infection, and **n**eoplasia (XMEN) disease

5. Hermansky-Pudlak syndrome is characterized by oculocutaneous albinism and platelet storage pool deficiency.

Q. Which of the following is not a usual clinical feature of HLH:

1. Splenomegaly
2. Hypertriglyceridemia
3. Increased ferritin levels
4. Decreased soluble CD25 levels

Answer: Decreased soluble CD25 levels

In fact, the soluble CD25 levels are elevated in HLH.

HLH patients have a constellation of symptoms and signs and that's why diagnosis is often delayed or missed, because these symptoms are present in many conditions, both common and rare.

Hemophagocytosis is present in 82 percent of patients. Markers of macrophage activity are increased and NK cell activity is low or absent (as we have already discussed in the question about pathogenesis).

Q. Which of the following laboratory abnormality is not typical for HLH:
    1. Anemia
    2. Thrombocytopenia
    3. Leukopenia
    4. All of the above are characteristic for HLH

Answer: leukopenia

HLH characteristically has bicytopenia: anemia and thrombocytopenia.

Q. The most common malignancy related to HLH is:
    1. Lymphoma

2. Leukemia
3. Plasma cell disorders
4. Solid childhood cancers

Answer: lymphoma

Q. The most common rheumatologic disorder associated with HLH is:
   1. Systemic juvenile idiopathic arthritis
   2. Adult onset rheumatoid arthritis
   3. Polyarteritis nodosa
   4. Juvenile Sjogren syndrome

Answer: Systemic juvenile idiopathic arthritis

It is also known as Still's disease.

HLH may develop any time during the course of a rheumatologic disorder.

Q. Apart from complete blood count, liver function tests, serum ferritin and triglyceride levels, bone marrow evaluation should be done in:
   1. Patients having cytopenias
   2. Patients having normal ferritin levels
   3. In cases of diagnostic dilemma
   4. In all patients regardless of other test results

Answer: In all patients regardless of other test results

All patients should have a bone marrow aspirate and biopsy to evaluate the cause of cytopenias and/or detect hemophagocytosis.

Bone marrow is infiltrated with macrophages in HLH and in majority of cases hemophagocytosis may also be seen but it must be noted that hemophagocytosis is **not** pathognomonic for HLH.

Q. Which of the following finding is not consistent with HLH:
   1. Elevated soluble IL-2R
   2. Reduced NK function
   3. Increased cell surface expression of CD107 alpha
   4. Reduced perforin

Answer: Increased cell surface expression of CD107 alpha

In fact, the level of cell surface expression of CD107 alpha are reduced, which reflect reduced NK function.

Level of sIL-2R correlate most closely with disease activity.

Q. Genetic testing for HLH is indicated in which patients:

1. In all patients who meet the diagnostic criteria for HLH
2. In all patients with a high likelihood of HLH based on the initial evaluation
3. Both of the above
4. It is not indicated except as a part of a clinical trial

Answer: both of the above

For genetic testing of HLH, next generation sequencing or whole exome sequencing are preferred. Sometimes intronic sequencing may be needed.

Q. The currently accepted diagnostic criteria for HLH are based on which trial:

1. HLH-2014
2. HLH-2004
3. HLH-1994
4. HLH-2018

Answer: HLH-2004

The diagnostic criteria for HLH:

1. In children and adults presence HLH mutations like *PRF1*, *UNC13D*, *STX11*, *STXBP2*, *Rab27A*, *SH2D1A*, *BIRC4*, *LYST*, *ITK*, *SLC7A7*, *XMEN*, *HPS* or other genes related to im-

mune regulation is diagnostic. In adults, an added condition is that along with heterozygosity of one of these genes, some clinical feature should also be present.

OR

Five of the following eight:

    a. Fever ≥38.5°C

    b. Splenomegaly

    c. Peripheral blood cytopenia, with at least two of the following: hemoglobin <9 g/dL (for infants <4 weeks, hemoglobin <10 g/dL); platelets <100,000/microL; absolute neutrophil count <1000/microL

    d. Hypertriglyceridemia (fasting triglycerides >265 mg/dL) and/or hypofibrinogenemia (fibrinogen <150 mg/dL)

    e. Hemophagocytosis in bone marrow, spleen, lymph node, or liver

    f. Low or absent NK cell activity

    g. Ferritin >500 ng/mL (the author prefers to consider a ferritin >3000 ng/mL as more indicative of HLH)

    h. Elevated soluble CD25 (soluble IL-2 receptor alpha [sIL-2R]) two standard deviations above age-adjusted laboratory-specific norms

It should be noted here that the above mentioned criteria are not exhaustive and in a rare disease such as HLH, institutional practices and personal clinical experience plays a big role in diagnosis. You may come across different sets of diagnostic criteria and to follow them would not be wrong.

Q. Which of the following is incorrect about HLH management:
1. A period of observation is justified in most pediatric patients, as the disease runs a self-limiting course
2. The HLH-94 consists induction chemo with etoposide and dexamethasone. Intrathecal methotrexate and hydrocortisone are given to those with central nervous system disease
3. After induction, patients who are recovering are weaned off therapy
4. After induction if the patient is not responding then allogeneic hematopoietic cell transplantation is performed

Answer: A period of observation is justified as in most pediatric patients, the disease runs a self-limiting course

HLH is a fulminant disease and treatment should be promptly initiated in most of the patients. That being said, if a patient is clinically stable and the ferritin is consistently below 10,000 ng/mL or rises from 1000 to 3000 ng/mL with only slightly elevated D-dimer and liver enzymes, many hematologists don't start treatment.

It goes without saying that if another disease is suspected underlying HLH (secondary HLH), then treatment of that disease should be initiated and in such cases HLH-94 protocol may not necessarily be followed.

The above mentioned treatment protocol is based on the HLH-94 trial, and another trial came later, known as the HLH-2004 trial which modified previous protocol by adding cyclosporine to the induction phase.

Q. Which of the following markers is not used for monitoring disease activity and/or response to treatment in cases of HLH:
1. Soluble IL-2 receptor alpha [sCD25]
2. Soluble hemoglobin-haptoglobin scavenger receptor [sCD163]
3. Ferritin
4. Bone marrow hemophagocytic count and ratio

Answer: Bone marrow hemophagocytic count and ratio

Q. The drug of choice for EBV induced HLH is:
1. Entecavir

2. Ritonavir
3. Rituximab
4. Ribavirin plus interferon-alpha

Answer: rituximab

IVIG is recommended as the drug of choice by some experts but the overall consensus is that rituximab is a more effective option.

Q. Which of the following is not an indication of allogeneic HCT in HLH:
1. Homozygous or compound heterozygous HLH gene mutations
2. Lack of response to initial HLH therapy
3. Central nervous system (CNS) involvement
4. Severe rheumatologic disorder

Answer: Severe rheumatologic disorder

The fourth indication of allo-HCT is hematologic malignancy.

Q. In patients of HLH who fail on initial HLH directed therapy as well as allo-HCT, the drug of choice is:
1. Alemtuzumab
2. Emapalumab
3. Etanercept

4. Abatacept

Answer: emapalumab

Emapalumab is an interferon gamma blocking anti-body and it is used in combination with dexamet-hasone.

Alemtuzumab plus etoposide is also an option but is not preferred.

LANGERHANS CELL HISTIOCYTOSIS (LCH)

Q. LCH is derived from:
1. Myeloid progenitor cells from the bone marrow
2. Langerhans cells of the skin
3. Both of the above
4. None of the above

Answer: Myeloid progenitor cells from the bone marrow

LCH is a clonal myeloid malignancy.

There were many historical "names" for this disorder, like histiocytosis-X, Letterer-Siwe disease, Hand-Schüller-Christian disease etc.

The name eosinophilic granuloma is sometimes still used to describe an individual lesion.

Q. Erdheim-Chester disease comes under which category of disorders, as per Histiocyte society:
1. C
2. L

3. R
4. M

Answer: L

The 5 categories of disorders in the Histiocyte society classification are:

1. L (Langerhans) group: LCH, indeterminate cell histiocytosis, Erdheim-Chester Disease (ECD), mixed LCH/ECD, and extracutaneous juvenile xanthogranuloma.
2. C (cutaneous and mucocutaneous) group: juvenile xanthogranuloma, adult xanthogranuloma, and cutaneous Rosai-Dorfman disease.
3. R (Rosai-Dorfman disease) group: Rosai-Dorfman disease and miscellaneous non-cutaneous histiocytosis.
4. M (malignant histiocytosis) group: includes histiocytosis secondary to malignant disorders.
5. H (hemophagocytic lymphohistiocytosis) group: primary and secondary hemophagocytic lymphohistiocytosis (HLH) and macrophage activation syndromes.

Q. LCH occurs most commonly in which age group:
1. 1-3 years
2. 3-6 years
3. 6-18 years

4. 18-24 years

Answer: 1-3 years

BRAF V600E mutation is commonly found in LCH cases.

Q. Acute disseminated, multisystem LCH is most commonly seen in:
1. Children less than three years old
2. Children more than three years old
3. Late adolescence and adults
4. Elderly population

Answer: children less than three years old

A more indolent disease involving a single organ is more common in older children and adults.

Q. Involvement of which of the following organs by LCH imparts the least risk compared to other organs mentioned below:
1. Liver
2. Hematopoietic system
3. Spleen
4. Lung

Answer: lung

In LCH, if certain organs are involved by the disease, prognosis will be worse. These organs are known as "risk organs" and include the hematopoietic system, liver, and/or spleen and denote a worse prognosis. Although the lung has been considered a "risk organ," more recent studies have suggested that it has less of an effect on prognosis.

Q. In adults, the most commonly affected bones by LCH are:

1. Jaws
2. Skull
3. Femur
4. Vertebra

Answer: jaws

The most frequent bony site of involvement in children is skull and in adults it is jaws, followed by the skull.

Q. Congenital self-healing reticulohistiocytosis is characteristically seen in:

1. LCH
2. MAS
3. Fabry's disease
4. Juvenile rheumatoid arthritis

Answer: LCH

It is the most common cutaneous manifestation of LCH along with an eczematous rash.

Q. Which is the most common endocrine abnormality encountered in:
1. Diabetes insipidus
2. Diabetes mellitus
3. Acromegaly
4. Cushing's syndrome

Answer: diabetes insipidus

Q. The nucleus in the abnormal cells in LCH characteristically resemble which shape:
1. Twisted towel
2. Pillared hall
3. Raindrop
4. Blurred glass

Answer: twisted towel

The nucleus is sometimes may also be described as having a coffee bean appearance.

It should not be confused with the shape of the Birbeck granules, also seen in LCH, which is described as a tennis racket.

Note that identification of Birbeck granules is done by electron microscopy.

Q. LCH cells express all of the following markers except:
1. CD1a
2. S100
3. CD207
4. CD107

Answer: CD107

CD207 is also known as langerin.

Q. Which of the following is not true about LCH:
1. Diagnosis is often established by biopsy of an osteolytic bone lesion or skin lesion and at the time of biopsy, a wide excision should be performed
2. Biopsy of the pituitary gland is required in cases with isolated pituitary involvement and in challenging cases identification of *BRAF* V600E in the peripheral blood or cerebrospinal fluid can support the diagnosis
3. In patients with isolated pituitary disease in whom biopsy in not possible, empiric chemotherapy may be started based on MRI findings
4. A light microscopy exam showing Langerhans cells is not sufficient and their iden-

tity must be confirmed either by positive immunohistochemical staining for CD1a and CD207 or by the identification of Birbeck granules by electron microscopy

Answer: Diagnosis is often established by biopsy of an osteolytic bone lesion or skin lesion and at the time of biopsy, a wide excision should be performed

While it's true that diagnosis is often established by biopsy of an osteolytic bone lesion or skin lesion and but at the time of biopsy, a wide excision should **NOT** be performed as LCH bone lesions will have complete or near complete healing with curettage alone or chemotherapy.

Q. In which patient population of LCH is pulmonary involvement more common:
  1. Male infants
  2. Adult males
  3. Female infants
  4. Adult females

Answer: adult males

Lung involvement occurs in approximately 10 percent of cases. It is less frequent in children than in adults, in whom smoking is a key etiologic factor. So lung involvement is more common in smoker adult population. In the affected patients high-resolution computed tomography (CT) scan reveals cysts and nodules characteristic of LCH.

Q. Involvement of which of the following bones by LCH will not come under "CNS-risk" lesions category:
  1. Facial bones
  2. Bones of anterior cranial fossa
  3. Bones of middle cranial fossa
  4. Bones of posterior cranial fossa

Answer: bones of posterior cranial fossa

Q. Which of the following is not a part of the triad of Hand-Schüller-Christian disease:
  1. Exophthalmos
  2. Diabetes insipidus
  3. Skull lesions
  4. Hepatosplenomegaly

Answer: hepatosplenomegaly

Another disease of the same groups as HSCD is Letterer-Siwe disease in which the findings are: lymphadenopathy, skin rash, hepatosplenomegaly, fever, anemia, and thrombocytopenia.

LCH of the bone (also known as eosinophilic granuloma of bone or histiocytosis X) is the third disease of this group.

Q. All of the following are correct about LCH of the bone except:
1. The most common age of presentation is 5 to 10 years
2. Monostotic bone lesion is more common than polyostotic bone lesions
3. Skull is the most commonly involved site in children and parietal bone is the most commonly affected bone
4. In adults the most common primary site of bone involvement is jaw

Answer: Skull is the most commonly involved site in children and parietal bone is the most commonly affected bone

While it's true that skull is the most common site in children but the most commonly involved bone of the skull is the frontal bone.

Q. The lesions of LCH are the least common in which part of the bone:
1. Diaphysis
2. Metaphysis
3. Epiphysis
4. The lesions are almost equally distributed

throughout the bone

Answer: epiphysis

The lesions are mostly found in the diaphysis or metaphysis.

When LCH involves the vertebrae, in extreme cases there may be flattening of vertebra, that has a "coin on edge" appearance, also known as vertebra plana.

Q. On radionuclide bone scans, LCH typically is:
1. Hot
2. Cold
3. Normal
4. Not identified

Answer: hot

Q. Which of the following is not true about treatment of LCH:
1. Almost all patients with osseous LCH are ultimately cured of their disease
2. LCH of bone is most commonly treated with curettage and a clean margin is not required for treatment
3. LCH lesions of the spine often involve the endochondral ossification centers, therefore reconstruction is a must

4. High risk LCH patients should be treated with 12 months of vinblastine and prednisone as per the LCH-III protocol

Answer: LCH lesions of the spine often involve the endochondral ossification centers, therefore reconstruction is a must

In fact, LCH lesions of the spine **do not** involve the endochondral ossification centers.

To clarify the first option, we must understand that while almost all of the patients with LCH of the bone will be cured but that doesn't mean that there are no recurrences; in fact, the recurrences are frequent.

If a question is asked about the role of radiation in LCH, then it will obviously depend on the clinical context. But to give a generalized view, radiation is not an initial or preferred approach and it is used in patients who recur despite repeated surgeries and/or chemo and in whom further surgery or chemo will not be of any benefit, as decided by the tumor board.

ERDHEIM-CHESTER DISEASE (ECD)

Q. Erdheim-Chester disease (ECD) is a:
1. Langerhans histiocytic disorder
2. Non-Langerhans histiocytic disorder
3. It's a mixed Langerhans and non-Langerhans histiocytic disorder
4. None of the above

Answer: non-Langerhans histiocytic disorder

This disorder arises from monocyte-macrophage lineage.

Q. ECD is characterized by:
1. Multifocal osteosclerotic lesions of the long bones
2. Multifocal osteosclerotic lesions of the short bones
3. Multifocal osteolytic lesions of the long bones
4. Multifocal osteolytic lesions of the short bones

Answer: Multifocal osteosclerotic lesions of the long bones

Q. The most common age of presentation of ECD is:
1. Children upto 4 years
2. Early adolescence
3. 50-60 years
4. More than 80 years

Answer: 50-60 years

Q. Touton cells are seen in which disorder:
1. Erdheim-Chester disease
2. Hemophagocytic lymphohistiocytosis
3. Langerhans cell histiocytosis
4. None of the above

Answer: Erdheim-Chester disease

Touton cells are multinucleated giant cells

Q. ECD cells express all of the following markers except:
1. CD68
2. CD163
3. Factor XIIIa
4. S100

Answer: S100

ECD cells don't express CD1a or S100, which are markers of LCH.

BRAF V600E mutation is found in about half of the patients with ECD.

Notes:
Treatment of ECD is not always indicated, the usual indications of for beginning treatment are:
1. Symptomatic disease
2. Evidence of organ dysfunction
3. CNS involvement, either symptomatic or asymptomatic
4. Evidence of organ dysfunction, or impending organ dysfunction

Q. Which of the following is not an initial treatment option for ECD:
1. Vemurafenib
2. Interferon alfa
3. Cladribine
4. Glucocorticoids

Answer: cladribine

In patients with BRAF V600E mutation, vemurafenib is the preferred initial treatment option, whereas in patients lacking this mutation interferon is the drug of choice. Some patients can't tolerate either of these therapies, in such patients glucocorticoids alone may be used.

Cladribine and cyclophosphamide are second line options.
MEK inhibitors, cobimetinib and trametinib are also options for the second line or later line of therapy.

It should be noted here that there is no known cure for ECD and with currently available therapies, the 5 year OS is about 70%.

Q. Enlargement of which of the following lymph nodes is always pathological:
     1. Inguinal
     2. Left supraclavicular
     3. Epitrochlear
     4. Suboccipital

Answer: epitrochlear

CONGENITAL NEUTROPENIA

Notes on clues obtained by physical examination that point to the underlying disorder leading to congenital neutropenia (note that the final diagnosis is dependent on the genetic testing, as many of the physical examination findings overlap):

1. Oculocutaneous albinism, peripheral neuropathy, and large granules in leukocytes – Chediak-Higashi syndrome
2. Metaphyseal dysplasia, pancreatic insufficiency – Shwachman-Diamond syndrome
3. Oculocutaneous albinism – Griscelli syndrome, Hermansky-Pudlak syndrome, p14 deficiency
4. Warts – WHIM syndrome (warts, hypogammaglobulinemia, infections, myelokathexis syndrome)
5. Hypoglycemia, growth retardation, hepatomegaly – Glycogen storage disease IB
6. Short-limbed short stature, hypoplastic hair – Cartilage hair hypoplasia
7. Skeletal myopathy, dilated cardiomyopathy – Barth's syndrome
8. Hypotonia, microcephaly, intellectual disability – Cohen syndrome

Q. Which of the following is not true about severe congenital neutropenia:

1. The most common mutation leading to SCN occurs in the *ELANE* gene and is transmitted as an autosomal dominant condition
2. In Kostmann syndrome, patients have mutations in *HAX1* with X-linked inheritance
3. In the Wiskott-Aldrich syndrome mutations is the WASP gene are seen
4. None of the above

Answer: In Kostmann syndrome, patients have mutations in *HAX1* with X-linked inheritance

While it's true that in Kostmann syndrome, patients have mutations in *HAX1* but the inheritance is autosomal recessive.

Q. Which of the following is not a part of the triad of Shwachman-Diamond syndrome:

1. Neutropenia
2. Metaphyseal dysplasia
3. Pancreatic insufficiency
4. Hyperglycemia

Answer: hyperglycemia

Q. Leukocyte adhesion deficiency is a cause of leukocytosis, which of the following is responsible for LAD II:

1. Defects of CD18
2. Lack of sialyl Lewis X
3. Excess of sialyl Lewis X
4. None of the above

Answer: lack of sialyl Lewis X

There are three types of LAD. Type I is associated with defects of CD18, type II is associated with lack of sialyl Lewis X.

Q. Chronic neutrophilic leukemia (CNL) is associated with

1. Activating germline mutation in *CSF3R*
2. Deactivating germline mutation in *CSF3R*
3. Activating somatic mutation in *CSF3R*
4. Deactivating somatic mutation in *CSF3R*

Answer: Activating germline mutation in *CSF3R*,

Notes: Infants with Down syndrome (trisomy of chromosome 21) may have a transient abnormal myelopoiesis (also called transient myeloproliferative disorder [TMD] of Down syndrome) that resembles congenital acute leukemia or chronic myeloid leukemia. TMD may resolve spontaneously, but evolves into overt acute myeloid leukemia in a subset of patients.

DRUG-INDUCED NEUTROPENIA
AND IMMUNE NEUTROPENIA

Q. Which of the following is not a risk factor for agranulocytosis:
1. Increasing age
2. Male gender
3. Renal failure
4. Underlying autoimmune disease

Answer: male gender

Agranulocytosis is more common in females.

An interesting risk factor is the combined use of ACE inhibitors and interferon.

Notes:
The list of drugs causing agranulocytosis is very long. The most important drugs that we should remember are: methimazole, carbimazole, sulfasalazine, trimethoprim-sulfamethoxazole, dipyrone combined with analgesics, clomipramine, and clozapine.

Q. Neonatal isoimmune neutropenia is more com-

monly caused by:
1. IgG antibodies to neutrophil-specific antigens inherited from the father
2. IgG antibodies to neutrophil-specific antigens inherited from the mother
3. IgM antibodies to neutrophil-specific antigens inherited from the father
4. IgM antibodies to neutrophil-specific antigens inherited from the mother

Answer: IgG antibodies to neutrophil-specific antigens inherited from the father

The prognosis of this disorder is good and apart from prophylactic antibiotics to prevent neonatal sepsis, nothing much needs to be done.

Q. Pure white cell aplasia is most often associated with:
1. Thymoma
2. Lymphoma
3. Small cell lung cancer
4. Non-small cell lung cancer

Answer: thymoma

Thymectomy and immunosuppressive therapy are used in this disorder.

Note that thymoma is also associated with pure red

cell aplasia.

Q. Which of the following is not true about infections and neutropenia:

1. Leukopenia with neutropenia is seen in approximately 25 to 50 percent of adults with typhoid fever
2. Neutropenia occurs in 20 to 30 percent of adults and children with brucellosis
3. Lymphopenia is seen in up to 87 percent patients of tuberculosis with varying degrees of neutropenia
4. Leukopenia occurs in approximately 25 percent of patients with rickettsialpox

Answer: Leukopenia occurs in approximately 25 percent of patients with rickettsialpox

In fact, leukopenia is seen in almost 75% of the patients.

CLONAL HEMATOPOIESIS OF INDETERMINATE POTENTIAL (CHIP), IDIOPATHIC AND CLONAL CYTOPENIAS OF UNCERTAIN SIGNIFICANCE (ICUS AND CCUS)

Q. An individual hematopoietic stem cell would be expected to contribute to approximately what percent of blood cell production:

1. 0.001
2. 0.01
3. 0.1
4. 1.0

Answer: 0.001%

Q. Which is the least commonly involved single gene mutation in CHIP:

1. *DNMT3A*
2. *TET2*
3. *ASXL1*
4. *TP53*

Answer: *TP53*

Q. In which of the following situations, testing to exclude a germline mutation in a cases of CHIP is not warranted:

1. Variant allele frequency 40 to 60 percent for mutations of *RUNX1*
2. Variant allele frequency 40 to 60 percent for mutations of *GATA2*
3. Variant allele frequency 20 percent or more for mutations of *DDX41*
4. Variant allele frequency 20 percent or more for mutations of *TP53*

Answer: Variant allele frequency 20 percent or more for mutations of *DDX41*

For DDX41 too, the variant allele frequency should be 40-60% to warrant germline mutation testing.

Genes like *DNMT3A, TET2, ASXL1* are not known to be inherited, and it is not necessary to exclude germline transmission if these mutations are identified with any frequency.

Q. Which of the following does not come under the definition of CHIP:

1. Variant allele frequency (VAF) ≥2 percent of an acquired mutation of a leukemia-associated gene

    2. The most common mutations affect *DN-MT3A*, *TET2*, and/or *ASXL1*

    3. Abnormal peripheral blood counts

    4. No clinical or pathologic evidence for a World Health Organization defined hematologic malignancy neoplasm

Answer: Abnormal peripheral blood counts

In fact, the peripheral blood counts should be normal.

If peripheral blood counts are not normal then the diagnosis in such cases will be clonal cytopenia of uncertain significance (CCUS).

It should be noted that modest levels of bone marrow dysplasia don't exclude the diagnosis of CHIP but if ≥10 percent of peripheral blood cells or bone marrow nucleated cells exhibit dysplasia, the condition should be classified as myelodysplastic syndrome (MDS).

Another related disorder is ARCH (aging related clonal hematopoiesis).

Q. The preferred method of testing for clonal hematopoiesis is:

    1. Next-generation sequencing (NGS)

    2. Flow cytometry

3. Karyotype combined with FISH
4. Proteomics analysis

Answer: next-generation sequencing (NGS)

A panel of leukemia-associated genes on peripheral blood or bone marrow are used for NGS.

Notes on diagnostic criteria for ICUS:
1. Cytopenia in one or more blood lineages that remain unexplained despite appropriate evaluation
2. No evidence of clonal hematopoiesis (CH); if a leukemia-associated mutation is detected, the variant allele frequency (VAF) should be <2 percent
3. No other evidence of a hematologic malignancy, according to World Health Organization (WHO) criteria. Note that there should be no dysplasia and if dysplasia is there in either peripheral blood or bone marrow, it should be less than 10%

Notes on diagnostic criteria for CCUS:
1. Unexplained, clinically meaningful cytopenias
2. CH is detected with ≥2 percent VAF of a leukemia-associated gene
3. No other evidence of a hematologic malignancy, as described above

Q. The risk of progression to MDS of leukemias is more in:

    1. ICUS

    2. CCUS

    3. The risk is similar in these two conditions

    4. There is no risk of progression in either ICUS or CCUS

Answer: CCUS

It is so because CCUS is associated with more mutations than ICUS (read the diagnostic criteria for these conditions carefully).

RECOMBINANT HEMATOPOIETIC GROWTH FACTORS

Notes, clinical uses of HGFs:

1. Transient bone marrow failure following chemotherapy
2. Hematopoietic stem cell and progenitor cell mobilization
3. Recovery from hematopoietic cell transplantation
4. Myelodysplastic syndromes
5. Aplastic anemia
6. Some forms of neutropenia
7. Inherited bone marrow failure syndromes
8. Human immunodeficiency virus (HIV) infection-associated neutropenia
9. Chronic anemias (eg, renal failure, prematurity, chronic disease/inflammation, HIV infection)
10. ITP and chemotherapy induced thrombocytopenia

Q. Which of the following is not true about myeloid growth factors:

1. The recommended dose of G-CSF is 5 mcg/kg per day for most clinical situations and

   10 mcg/kg per day for peripheral blood stem cell mobilization
2. The recommended dose of GM-CSF is 250 mcg/m2 per day
3. G-CSF is usually started within 24 hours after administration of chemotherapy
4. Following intravenous bolus injection, both GM-CSF and G-CSF induce a transient leukopenia in the first 30 minutes after administration

Answer: G-CSF is usually started within 24 hours after administration of chemotherapy

It must be understood that G-CSF is usually started **AFTER** at least 24 hours of chemotherapy.

Toxicities of myeloid growth factors:
1. Transient leukopenia
2. Flu-like symptoms
3. Bone pain, coincident with or shortly after administration
4. Increased risk of a therapy-related myeloid neoplasm
5. Pathogenic neutrophil infiltration (acute febrile neutrophilic dermatosis or Sweet syndrome) and cutaneous necrotizing vasculitis (leukocytoclastic vasculitis)
6. Capillary leak syndrome

Q. The most common side effect of erythropoietin is:

1. Hypertension
2. Flu-like syndrome
3. Deep venous thrombosis
4. Nephrotoxicity

Answer: hypertension

The drugs of choice for erythropoietin induced hypertension are beta-adrenergic blockers.

PROPHYLAXIS AND MANAGE-
MENT OF NEUTROPENIA

Q. The gold standard for determining the adequacy of the bone marrow's ability to produce neutrophils is:
  1. Neutrophil stress test
  2. Examination of a bone marrow
  3. Flow cytometry
  4. Functional oxidative stress assays

Answer: examination of the bone marrow

Q. Lymphocytopenia can occur in:
  1. HIV-AIDS
  2. Sepsis
  3. Postoperative period
  4. All of the above

Answer: all of the above

Indications for use of G-CSF in non-chemotherapy induced neutropenia:
  1. Severe congenital neutropenia
  2. Cyclic neutropenia
  3. Neutropenia associated with early

myeloid arrest
4. Acquired immune deficiency syndrome (AIDS)
5. Acquired bone marrow defects with severe neutropenia (ie, ANC < 500 cells/microL)
6. Chronic idiopathic neutropenia with severe neutropenia
7. Drug-induced neutropenia/agranulocytosis with severe neutropenia

Q. Granulocyte transfusions are more useful in patients with sepsis who have not shown a clinical response to antibiotics within 24 to 48 hours and the pathogens are:
1. Gram negative bacteria
2. Gram positive bacteria
3. Invasive infections
4. Mycobacterial infections (disseminated)

Answer: Gram positive bacteria

Notes on diseases of immune function that can be treated by hematopoietic stem cell transplant:
1. Severe combined immunodeficiency
2. Wiskott-Aldrich syndrome
3. CD40 ligand deficiency (X-linked hyper IgM syndrome)
4. CD40 deficiency (autosomal recessive hyper IgM syndrome)
5. X-linked lymphoproliferative disease

6. Interferon gamma receptor defects
7. NF kappa B essential modifier (NEMO) deficiency
8. Hemophagocytic lymphohistiocytosis
9. Chronic granulomatous disease
10. Leukocyte adhesion deficiency type 1
11. Griscelli syndrome type 2
12. Chediak-Higashi syndrome

Notes on CTCAE for hematologic toxicity:

NCI CTCAE (National Cancer Institute Common Terminology Criteria for Adverse Events) divides the categories of adverse effects in five grades, but note that it's not necessary for a toxicity to have 5 categories, sometimes it goes only up to grade 3.

1. Febrile neutropenia:
    a. There is no specified grade 1
    b. There is no specified grade 2
    c. Grade 3: ANC <1000/microL with a single temperature >38.3°C (100.4°F) or a sustained temperature ≥38°C (100°F) for more than one hour
    d. Grade 4: Life-threatening consequences; urgent intervention indicated
    e. Grade 5: death
2. Hemoglobin:
    a. Grade 1: <LLN to 10 g/dL
    b. Grade 2: 8 to 10 g/dL
    c. Grade 3: <8 g/dL
    d. Grade 4: Life-threatening conse-

quences; urgent intervention indicated
e. Grade 5: death
3. Neutrophils:
    a. Grade 1: <LLN to 1500/microL
    b. Grade 2: 1000 to 1500/microL
    c. Grade 3: 500 to 1000/microL
    d. Grade 4: <500/microL
    e. There is no specified grade 5
4. lymphocytes:
    a. Grade 1: <LLN to 800/microL
    b. Grade 2: 500 to 800/microL
    c. Grade 3: 200 to 500/microL
    d. Grade 4: <200/microL
    e. There is no specified grade 5
5. CD4 count:
    a. Grade 1: <LLN to 500/microL
    b. Grade 2: 200 to 500/microL
    c. Grade 3: 50 to 200/microL
    d. Grade 4: <50/microL
    e. There is no specified grade 5
6. Platelets:
    a. Grade 1: <LLN to 75,000/microL
    b. Grade 2: 50000 to 75000/microL
    c. Grade 3: 25000 to 50000/microL
    d. Grade 4: <25000/microL
    e. There is no specified grade 5

Q. Antimicrobial prophylaxis is generally not indicated in which patients of chemotherapy induced neutropenia:

1. Patients who are expected to be neutro-penic with ANC <1500/microL for >7 days
2. Patients with neutropenia and ongoing comorbidities
3. Patients with neutropenia with significant hepatic or renal dysfunction regardless of duration of neutropenia
4. Antimicrobial prophylaxis is indicated in all of the above mentioned situations

Answer: Patients who are expected to be neutro-penic with ANC <1500/microL for >7 days

Antimicrobial prophylaxis is indicated in patients of chemotherapy induced neutropenia who are at high risk of infectious complications, e.g.

1. Those who are expected to be neutropenic (ANC <500 cells/microL) for >7 days
2. Patients with neutropenic fever who have ongoing comorbidities regardless of the duration of neutropenia
3. Those having evidence of significant hep-atic or renal dysfunction regardless of the duration of neutropenia
4. Those undergoing allogeneic HCT
5. Neutropenic patients receiving induction chemotherapy for acute leukemia

By contrast, low-risk patients are those in whom the duration of neutropenia (ANC <500 cells/microL) is expected to be less than seven days and who have no comorbidities and no evidence of significant hepatic or renal dysfunction and in these patients antimicrobial prophylaxis is not indicated regardless of ANC.

Q. The preferred drug for antimicrobial prophylaxis in chemotherapy induced neutropenic patients at high-risk of infectious complications is:
1. Levofloxacin
2. Azithromycin
3. Carbapenems
4. Aztreonam

Answer: levofloxacin

The timing for initiating levofloxacin is not very clear but most of the times it's started on the day or the day after administration of chemotherapy and continued till neutropenia has resolved or if the patient becomes febrile, because if the patient becomes febrile then empiric antibacterial regimen should be initiated and levofloxacin should be discontinued.

Another drug still in use and extensively studied is ciprofloxacin. It has greater in vitro activity than levofloxacin against *P. aeruginosa*, but levofloxacin has greater in vitro activity against gram-positive bacteria (eg, alpha-hemolytic streptococci) and is given only once daily compared with twice daily for ciprofloxacin. So these factors make levofloxacin a better drug.

Prolongation of the QT interval is a problematic side effect of quinolones and should be watched out for, especially if the patient is also receiving another drug that causes QT prolongation.

TMP-SMX was used in the past but it's no longer used due to its lack of activity against P. aeruginosa.

Q. The IDSA guidelines recommend that the prophylactic use of colony stimulating factors should be considered for afebrile patients in whom the anticipated risk of fever and neutropenia is:
1. ≥10%
2. ≥20%
3. ≥30%
4. In all patients regardless of the risk of fever and neutropenia

Answer: ≥20%

Please remember this number.

Notes on patients with chemotherapy-induced neutropenic fever who are at high risk for serious complications:
If a patient has any of the following characteristics then he will be considered at high risk:
1. Receipt of cytotoxic therapy sufficiently

myelosuppressive to result in anticipated severe neutropenia (ANC <500 cells/mcL) for >7 days
2. MASCC risk index score <21
3. CISNE score of ≥3
4. Alemtuzumab use within the past two months
5. Uncontrolled or progressive cancer
6. Hepatic or renal insufficiency
7. Presence of uncontrolled comorbid conditions

Q. The term neutrophilia refers to what:
1. ANC >7700/microL
2. Total leukocyte count >11000/microL
3. ANC >4500/microL
4. ANC >10000/microL

Answer: ANC >7700/microL

Glucocorticoids lead to release of granulocytes from the bone marrow and are associated with neutrophilia.

Q. Fever in neutropenic patients is defined as:
1. A single oral temperature of ≥38.3°C
2. A temperature of ≥38.0°C sustained over a one-hour period
3. A temperature of ≥100.4°F sustained over a

one-hour period
4. All of the above

Answer: all of the above

Q. Fever in a neutropenic patient should be considered a medical emergency and broad-spectrum antibacterials should be given:
1. Within 60 minutes of triage
2. Within 90 minutes of triage
3. After receiving blood culture reports
4. Not until the patient is hemodynamically stable

Answer: within 60 minutes of triage

Q. The most frequent pathogens identified during neutropenic fever episodes are:
1. Gram-positive bacteria
2. Gram-negative bacteria
3. Fungi
4. Viruses

Answer: Gram-positive bacteria

But it should be noted that the antibiotic coverage must be given for Gram-negative bacteria also because of their virulence and association with sepsis.

Q. Which of the following is not correct about the treatment of neutropenic fever:

1. Ceftazidime monotherapy should not be used when there is concern for a gram-negative infection
2. Antipseudomonal beta-lactam agent should be a part of the initial regimen
3. Vancomycin may be added to the initial regimen if hypotension, mental status changes, pneumonia or cellulitis are there
4. Anaerobic coverage should be added to the regimen if there is suspicion of neutropenic enterocolitis

Answer: Ceftazidime monotherapy should not be used when there is concern for a gram-negative infection

The fact is that Ceftazidime monotherapy should not be used when there is concern for a gram-**positive** infection because ceftazidime is not active against Gram-positive bacteria induced sepsis.

Antipseudomonal beta-lactam agents are: cefepime, meropenem, imipenem-cilastatin and piperacillin-tazobactam. As mentioned above ceftazidime monotherapy should not be used.

Notes about some key points in the management of neutropenic fever:

1. Monotherapy with the above mentioned beta-lactam agents generally demonstrated equivalent outcomes compared with two-drug regimens in clinical trials.
2. In a scenario where there is a high prevalence of multidrug-resistant gram-negative bacilli, initial empirical antibacterial therapy with piperacillin-tazobactam plus tigecycline may have some advantages over monotherapy.
3. Patients with a history of an immediate-type hypersensitivity reaction to penicillin should not receive beta-lactams or carbapenems.
4. Gram-positive bacteria targeting agents like vancomycin, are **not** recommended as a standard part of the initial regimen.
5. Gram-positive coverage should be added in patients with any of the following findings:
   a. Hemodynamic instability or other signs of severe sepsis
   b. Pneumonia
   c. Positive blood cultures for gram-positive bacteria
   d. Suspected central venous catheter (CVC)-related infection
   e. Skin or soft tissue infection
   f. In patients with increased risk of *viridans* group streptococcal infections

Caution should be taken with certain combinations, e.g., the combination of vancomycin and piperacillin-tazobactam has been associated with acute kidney injury.

Prolonged use of vancomycin has been associated with vancomycin resistant enterococci.

Q. Empiric antifungal coverage should be considered in high-risk patients who have persistent fever after how many days of a broad-spectrum antibacterial regimen:
    1. 1-2
    2. 3-4
    3. 4-5
    4. More than 1 week

Answer: 4-5

The most correct answer is 4 days with the range being from 4 to 7 days.

Q. Which of the following drugs should be used for pneumonia caused by MRSA:
    1. Vancomycin
    2. Linezolid
    3. Daptomycin
    4. All of the above

Answer: either vancomycin or linezolid

For MRSA infections, three antibiotics are commonly used: vancomycin, linezolid and daptomycin. Out of these, daptomycin should not be used in patients with pneumonia because it does not achieve sufficiently high concentrations in the respiratory tract.

Q. What are the treatment options for vancomycin resistant enterococci:
  1. Linezolid
  2. Daptomycin
  3. Both of the above
  4. None of the above

Answer: both of the above

Q. The drug of choice for extended spectrum beta-lactamase producing Gram-negative bacilli is:
  1. Meropenem
  2. Vancomycin
  3. Linezolid
  4. Daptomycin

Answer: meropenem

Carbapenems, eg, imipenem, meropenem, are the drug of choice for ESBL producing Gram-negative bacilli.

Q. What are the treatment options for carbapene-mase-producing bacteria:
  1. Colistin
  2. Tigecycline
  3. Both of the above
  4. None of the above

Answer: both of the above

Q. In patients receiving fluconazole prophylaxis, which are the most likely causes of fungal infection:
  1. *Candida glabrata*
  2. *Candida krusei*
  3. *Aspergillus*
  4. All of the above

Answer: all of the above

Note that most of the Candida species are sensitive to fluconazole but glabrata and krusei are not.

Q. The 2010 IDSA guidelines for empiric antifungal therapy recommend all of the following as suitable empiric antifungal therapy except:
  1. Amphotericin B deoxycholate
  2. Caspofungin
  3. Itraconazole

4. Fluconazole

Answer: fluconazole

Other options are lipid formulations of amphotericin and voriconazole.

Notes that echinocandins (caspofungin) are not active against *Cryptococcus* spp, *Trichosporon* spp, and filamentous molds other than *Aspergillus* spp, such as *Fusarium* spp. They are also not active against the endemic fungi (*Histoplasma*, *Blastomyces*, *Coccidioides* spp).

Q. In cases of central venous catheter (CVC)-related infections, in addition to prompt initiation of antibiotics, CVC removal is recommended for patients with catheter-related bloodstream infections in which all of the following organisms except:
  1. S. aureus
  2. *P. aeruginosa*
  3. *Candida*
  4. Enterobacter

Answer: enterobacter

Other organisms which warrant the removal of CVC are rapidly growing nontuberculous mycobacteria.

Antibiotics should be administered for a minimum

of 14 days following catheter removal **and** clearance of blood cultures.

Other scenarios where removal of CVC is recommended are:
1. Tunnel infection
2. Port pocket infection
3. Septic thrombosis
4. Endocarditis
5. Sepsis with hemodynamic instability
6. Bloodstream infection that persists despite ≥72 hours of therapy with appropriate antibiotics

Note that for CVC -associated bacteremia caused by coagulase-negative staphylococci, the CVC may be retained.

Q. Which of the following strategies should be promptly used in all patients with established neutropenic fever:
1. Empiric antibiotics
2. G-CSF
3. Both of the above
4. None of the above

Answer: empiric antibiotics

This point should be clearly understood. According to the IDSA and other such guidelines, the use of colony stimulating factors is **NOT** recommended in all patients with established neutropenia and fever. They are indicated only in those patients who are at **high risk** of infectious complications.

Q. Which of the following is not correct:

1. Use of granulocyte-macrophage colony stimulating factor (GM-CSF) has been associated with a higher incidence of thrombocytopenia and other complications when given with concurrent chemoradiotherapy
2. G-CSF should be used cautiously, if at all, during concomitant chemoradiotherapy for head and neck cancer because it has been associated with reduced locoregional tumor control
3. Most of the guidelines have recommended against the use of CSFs in afebrile patients who have already developed severe neutropenia after chemotherapy
4. Use of CSFs is generally associated with significantly improved overall mortality and infection-related mortality as compared with antibiotics alone

Answer: Use of CSFs is generally associated with significantly improved overall mortality and infection-related mortality as compared with antibiotics alone

In fact, the use of CSFs is generally **NOT** associated with significantly improved overall mortality and infection-related mortality as compared with anti-biotics alone

Notes on dose and timing of G-CSF and GM-CSF:
1. The recommended dose of G-CSF (filgrastim, filgrastim-sndz, tbo-filgrastim) is 5 mcg/kg per day and for GM-CSF (sargramostim), 250 mcg/m2 per day.
2. Therapy is usually begun 24 to 72 hours after cessation of chemotherapy and is often continued with twice weekly monitoring of blood counts, until the ANC reaches 5000 to 10,000/microL.
3. Because of the potential sensitivity of rapidly dividing myeloid cells to cytotoxic chemotherapy, growth factors should be discontinued several days before the next chemotherapy treatment and they should not be given on the same day as chemotherapy.
4. Myelosuppression is more profound if the myeloid growth factors were given immediately prior to or on the same day as the chemotherapy.
5. The recommended dose of pegfilgrastim is 6 mg in adults and 100 mcg/kg [maximum 6 mg] in children and it is given 24 hours after chemotherapy.